Defeating Candida

Unlocking the Secrets of Vitality and Rediscovering Wellness

Rossana Lewis

TABLE OF CONTENT

Chapter 1: Candida 101

1.1 Exploring Candida: Causes and Symptoms

Candidiasis is a fungal infection caused by an overgrowth of a type of yeast that lives on your body (Candida albicans). A candidiasis infection often appears on your skin, vagina or mouth, where Candida naturally lives in small amounts. Healthy bacteria on your body prevent yeast overgrowth. Imagine you have a two-armed scale with healthy bacteria on one side and yeast on the other. The scale stays balanced until disruption occurs from stress, a poor diet, a weakened immune system or an uncontrolled medical condition. When something disrupts your scale, a Candidiasis infection occurs.

What Causes Candidiasis?

A candidiasis infection is the result of an overgrowth of Candida yeast due to an imbalance of healthy bacteria and yeast in your body. Triggers that disrupt the balance of bacteria and yeast include:

- Taking antibiotics, steroids, oral contraceptives, medicines that cause dry mouth or medicines that turn off healthy bacteria.
- Feeling stressed.
- Eating a diet high in refined carbohydrates, sugar or yeast.
- Having uncontrolled diabetes, HIV, cancer or a compromised immune system.
- Experiencing hormonal changes (pregnancy).

Symptoms of Candidiasis

Symptoms of candidiasis vary depending on the location of the infection. Symptoms of candidiasis include:

- Red patch of skin (rash) with small, raised bumps (pustules).
- Itching.
- Burning sensation.
- Vaginal discharge (white or yellow).
- White patches or sores in your mouth that cause loss of taste or pain when eating or swallowing.
- Swelling (inflammation).

1.2 Types of Candida Infections

Oral Thrush: If the candida yeast spreads to your mouth and throat, it can cause an infection called oral candidiasis, or oralthrush. It's most common in newborns, older adults, and people with weakened immune systems. You may be more likely to get it if you:

- Are being treated for cancer
- Take medications such as corticosteroids and wide-spectrum antibiotics
- Wear dentures
- Have diabetes

Symptoms of oral thrush include:

- White or yellow patches on your tongue, lips, gums, roof of your mouth, and inner cheeks
- Redness or soreness in your mouth and throat
- Cracking at the corners of your mouth
- Pain when swallowing, if it spreads to your throat

Vaginal Candidiasis: Three out of four people with vaginas will get at least one genital yeast infection during their lifetime. This happens when too much yeast grows in the vagina. (Men and those assigned male at birth can also get genital yeast infections, but it's much less common). A yeast infection typically happens when the balance in the vagina changes. This can be caused by:

- Pregnancy
- Diabetes
- Some medicines, including antibiotics and birth control pills
- Use of some douches, vaginal sprays, lubricants, or spermicides
- A weakened immune system

- Wearing a wet bathing suit or workout clothes, or underwear that doesn't breathe

Occasionally, the infection can be passed from person to person during sex.

The symptoms include:

- Extreme itchiness in the vagina
- Redness and swelling of the vagina and vulva (the outer part of the female genitals)
- Pain and burning when you urinate
- Discomfort during sex
- A thick, white "cottage cheese" discharge from the vagina

Because these symptoms can be similar to other infections such as bacterial vaginosis (bacterial overgrowth in the vagina) and sexually transmitted diseases, it's important to visit your doctor if you're experiencing them. Most times, an over-the-counter antifungal suppository, tablet, or cream will knock out the infection. Your doctor might also prescribe a single dose of a prescription antifungal medicine such as fluconazole. Tell your doctor if you get yeast infections more than four times a year. They may recommend regular doses of antifungal medication over several months to fight the repeated infections.

Candidiasis in Men: Candida can infect male genitals, too. That shouldn't be too surprising as the fungus that causes it is normally present on your skin. But men are more likely to get candidiasis on the head of their penis if they have sex with a partner with vaginal candidiasis.

Candidiasis of your penis is also more likely if you:

- Aren't circumcised
- Take antibiotics often
- Have diabetes
- Have a weakened immune system
- Are overweight
- Don't wash regularly

Symptoms include:

- Moist skin on your penis
- A white substance in your skin folds
- White or shiny skin
- Redness, itching, or burning

Cutaneous Candidiasis: "Cutaneous" means affecting the skin. So, any type of candidiasis on the surface of your skin falls into this type.

Candidiasis infections most likely occur in places that are warm and moist, including:

- Your armpits
- Your groin
- Your belly button
- Under your breasts
- The spaces between your fingers and toes
- Your genitals
- Any skin folds on your stomach

Conditions that make cutaneous candidiasis more likely include:

- Hot or humid weather
- Wearing tight or synthetic underwear or clothing
- Not washing enough
- Not changing underwear or diapers often enough

- Having a weak immune system
- Pregnancy
- Being overweight
- Taking antibiotics or other medicines
- Having other skin conditions, such as psoriasis

You can treat candidiasis on your skin by keeping the area as dry as you can. You also can use antifungal creams. Ask your doctor which is best depending on where your infection is. If you're otherwise healthy, your candidiasis should go away easily. You can also take steps to make your infection less likely to happen again.

Diaper Rash from Yeast Infection: Though diaper rash is usually caused by leaving a wet or soiled diaper on for too long, once your baby's skin is irritated, infection is more likely. If their diaper rash isn't going away, check if their bottom is red and sensitive, and if there's a raised red border around the sores. If so, have your pediatrician check for candidiasis. It can be treated with an antifungal cream. Keeping your baby's bottom clean and dry is a good start to help prevent diaper rash and candidiasis.

Invasive Candidiasis: If candida enters your bloodstream (usually through medical equipment or devices), it can travel to your heart, brain, blood, eyes, and bones. This can cause a serious, life-threatening infection called invasive candidiasis. People who have recently been admitted to a hospital or live in a healthcare facility, such as a nursing home, are most at risk. Like other types of yeast infections, your chances of getting invasive candidiasis are greater if you have diabetes, a weakened immune system, kidney failure, or are on antibiotics .

The symptoms include fever and chills. It can be hard to diagnose because it's likely that a person with this infection is already sick with another condition.

Invasive candidiasis is treated with an oral or intravenous dose of antifungal medication. If you are having surgery and have higher odds of a yeast infection, your doctor might prescribe a series of antifungal medicines before the procedure.

Chapter 2: Candida Overgrowth: Recognizing the Signs

2.1 Identifying Candida Overgrowth Symptoms

Candida overgrowth is one of the most common conditions especially among autoimmune patients. There are thousands of patients with digestive issues, fatigue, brain fog, recurring fungal infections, skin problems, mood swings, and more, all caused by Candida overgrowth. In your body, the good bacteria, bad bacteria and Candida (among other forms of yeast, viruses, and even mites) that make up your gut microbiome exist in a balanced state. In fact, your microbiome is like a rainforest, with many different species living together in harmony.

When one species gets out of balance in your rainforest, everything gets out of control. When this balance is tipped between Candida and other microorganisms, Candida overgrowth occurs. Candidiasis, or yeast overgrowth, is very common and causes Candida overgrowth symptoms such as bloating, constipation, rashes, fungal infections, fatigue, brain fog, and mood swings.

Because yeast overgrowth can become a full-body problem, Candida overgrowth symptoms can be experienced in many different forms nearly anywhere in the body.

Feeling Tired, Worn Down, or Suffering from Chronic Fatigue or Fibromyalgia: Gut infections such as Candida overgrowth can suppress the immune system and interfere with energy levels.

Furthermore, Candidiasis is often accompanied by nutrient deficiencies such as vitamin B6, essential fatty acids, and magnesium. Particularly, magnesium deficiency has been known to cause fatigue.

Digestive Issues Such as Bloating, Constipation, or Diarrhea: The excess Candida can begin a fermentation process in your gut that produces its own swelling and belly bloat, much like when bread rises. This happens because good bacteria are depleted due to the overgrown Candida in your microbiome. When your gut bacteria is imbalanced you can experience digestive issues which include constipation, diarrhea, nausea, gas, cramps, and bloating. Colon Comfort may help to regain regularity over your digestive tract and bowel movements.

Autoimmune Diseases such as Hashimoto's Thyroiditis, Rheumatoid Arthritis, Ulcerative Colitis, Lupus, Psoriasis, Scleroderma, or Multiple Sclerosis: Candida overgrowth damages your gut lining, which allows for toxins, microbes, protein, and undigested food particles to escape into your bloodstream. Your immune system marks these foreign invaders as pathogens and attacks them. As the invaders continue escaping, your immune system goes into overdrive, sending more antibodies to battle the invaders and inducing more inflammation.

Difficulty Concentrating, Poor Memory, Lack of Focus, ADD, ADHD, Irritability, Mood Swings, Anxiety, or Depression, and/or Brain Fog: Excess yeast coats the lining of your intestinal tract and suppresses your ability to make or secrete serotonin. Candidiasis also affects your brain and mood function by producing chemicals that are directly toxic to the brain such as canditoxin and acetaldehyde.

Skin Issues Including Eczema, Psoriasis, Hives, and Rashes: Once Candida cells escape into your bloodstream, they can colonize on your skin and result in skin issues such as eczema, psoriasis, and rashes. In fact, researchers have taken skin cultures of eczema patients and more often than not, yeast was found in the samples.

Vaginal Infections, Urinary Tract Infections, Rectal Itching, or Vaginal Itching: An overgrowth of Candida can lead to Candidiasis of the vagina, also known as a yeast infection. Yeast infections are extremely common. It's estimated that 75% of all women will get at least one vaginal yeast infection in their lifetime, and half of those will have at least one recurrence. Although it's much less common, urinary tract infections can also be a Candida symptom.

Severe Seasonal Allergies or Itchy Ears: Seasonal allergy symptoms are caused by your immune system responding to something in the environment, such as pollen in the air. However, the reason your responses to these environmental allergens are heightened is often that your immune system is on high alert due to gut infections such as Candida overgrowth.

Strong Sugar and Refined Carbohydrate Cravings: Because yeast feeds on carbohydrates, once you have a yeast overgrowth, the Candida will cause you to crave sugar, leading to a vicious cycle that's hard to break.

2.2 Effects on Digestion and Overall Health

Candida overgrowth doesn't confine its effects to one area; it can significantly impact digestion and overall well-being. Understanding these effects is very important in addressing candida-related issues. Let's have a look at how these overgrowth affect your body:

Digestive Discomfort: Candida overgrowth often manifests with digestive disturbances. Symptoms may include bloating, gas, abdominal pain, and irregular bowel movements. These disruptions can affect daily comfort and quality of life.

Leaky Gut Syndrome: The presence of candida can contribute to the development of leaky gut syndrome. This condition occurs when the intestinal barrier becomes compromised, allowing undigested food particles, toxins, and pathogens to pass through the intestinal lining and into the bloodstream, triggering various health issues.

Nutrient Absorption Impairment: As candida overgrowth compromises the gut lining, it can impair nutrient absorption. This leads to deficiencies in essential vitamins and minerals, affecting overall health and vitality.

Weakened Immune Response: The gut plays a pivotal role in the immune system. Candida overgrowth can disrupt this balance, leading to a weakened immune response. Individuals may experience frequent infections or find it challenging to fight off illnesses.

Fatigue and Cognitive Fog: Candida overgrowth can contribute to persistent fatigue and mental fog. The body's energy is diverted to combatting the overgrowth, leaving individuals feeling chronically fatigued. Brain fog, difficulty concentrating, and memory issues are also common complaints.

Skin and Oral Issues: Candida overgrowth can manifest externally, leading to skin problems such as rashes, itching, or oral thrush. These visible signs often hint at internal imbalances caused by candida.

Chapter 3: Holistic Approaches to Candida Treatment

3.1 Understanding Holistic Health in Candida Treatment

It's a mistake to treat Candida with antifungals (prescription or herbal medicines) and expect that it won't grow back. When working with Candida it's important to approach it from many angles, to ensure that you are healthy enough to resist another attempt to grow. Here are things you should focus on.

Test to Make Sure You Actually Have Candida: Don't assume you have Candida!! There are other gut bacteria and vaginal infections that can cause similar symptoms. It might sound obvious, however a lot of damage can be done to your healthy microbiome if you continue to take antifungals when you don't need to. Stool tests and vaginal microbiome tests are easy to do and will tell you if there are other fungi or bacteria that could be contributing to your problems. A test can tell you what type of Candida overgrowth you have, the common types are C. albicans and C. glabrata. The treatment for different strains of Candida can vary.

Address Lifestyle Factors that Encourage Candida Overgrowth: Lifestyle factors that allow Candida to flourish include diet choices, alcohol and stress. A low sugar/ low yeast/low alcohol diet is generally recommended for reducing the ability of Candida to reproduce. While you're reducing the sugary and processed foods, remember to increase your healthy foods. Foods such as garlic, herbs and vegetables contribute to a healthy microbiome, which will resist any overgrowth. Additionally, vaginal Candida can be passed back and forth between sexual partners, so vaginal and oral hygiene is important, as well as making sure your partner is treated too!

Support Your Immune System: When Candida becomes overgrown, it could be a sign of a low immune response. It's important to explore this and determine if you need to support your immune system during your treatment.

Support Your Hormones: One of the most common mistakes in women with recurrent Candida is that they have high estrogen levels that haven't been addressed. Candida flourishes in a high estrogen environment (this is why Candida is not common after menopause). It's very helpful to look at your hormonal signs and symptoms. If you have heavy bleeding; fibroids; endometriosis; bloating or migraines before a period, it could be a red flag to let us know that your hormone imbalance could be driving the Candida. Are your Candida symptoms worse around ovulation or before a period? If hormones are not addressed, then the Candida has a high chance of growing back.

Investigate Digestion: Candida overgrowth in the digestive system can be due to low stomach acid allowing fungus and yeast to flourish. Bacteria such as Helicobacter pylori can create an environment in which Candida can thrive. So investigating which bugs are in your digestive system can be one of the keys to eradicating it. Constipation may also contribute to Candida problems if your body is not allowing Candida to be eliminated. If you have a lot of digestive problems such as bloating, nausea, reflux, fullness after eating and constipation, your naturopath might investigate SIFO (small intestine fungal overgrowth). SIFO is similar to SIBO however with a Candida overgrowth in the small intestine as well as bacteria. Candida overgrowth is also a known cause of leaky gut. If your digestive system is more permeable than it should be, it's possible for the Candida (and bacteria) to travel into the bloodstream and into circulation. Once in circulation, Candida can cause immune activation, widespread inflammation and symptoms such as diarrhea.

Investigate Triggers for Candida Overgrowth: A common trigger for recurrent Candida overgrowth is the use of antibiotics for acute conditions such as urinary tract infections or sinus infections. If this sounds like you, please seek help from your naturopath to address these infections without resorting to antibiotics. Antibiotics destroy healthy gut bacteria and allow Candida to overgrow.

Treat the Candida Until it's Gone: Many women are so relieved when they first start to experience a few days without Candida symptoms that they get excited and assume that it's gone for good. Candida is a stubborn fungal overgrowth and in my experience can take around 12 weeks for it to shift. All the other factors described above need to have been addressed before you can feel confident that it's gone. It's important to retest for Candida after 3 months of treatment and then enter into a period of 3 months of maintenance.

Restore Healthy Gut Bacteria and Vaginal Microbiome After Treatment: Have you been on a super strict Candida diet and thought you'd got rid of it at last? Only to have your Candida grow back as soon as you get stressed or have sex with a new partner? I can't stress enough how important this last step is! Failing to restore healthy microbiota is the number one reason why Candida can regrow after your treatment. If you go to all the effort and expense to rid yourself of Candida and you don't restore your healthy bacteria, then you are leaving the door open for Candida to come storming back. This final step involves eating plenty of fresh vegetables, taking appropriate probiotics and then testing to see if you have a good balance of healthy gut bacteria, or vaginal bacteria.

3.2 Balancing Diets, Lifestyle and Supplements

Treating candida involves a holistic approach that harmonizes diet, lifestyle, and targeted supplements. Here's how to effectively balance these elements to combat candida overgrowth:

Candida-Friendly Diet:

- Embrace an anti-candida diet rich in whole foods. Prioritize fiber, low-sugar fruits, vegetables, lean proteins, and healthy fats.
- Avoid sugar, refined carbohydrates, and processed foods that can feed candida growth.
- Consider incorporating natural antifungal foods like garlic, coconut oil, oregano, and ginger into your meals.

Lifestyle Adjustments:

- Manage stress through techniques like meditation, yoga, or deep breathing. Stress can weaken the immune system and exacerbate candida overgrowth.

- Regular exercise supports overall health and boosts immunity, aiding in candida control.

- Prioritize sufficient sleep to promote healing and support the body's natural defenses against candida.

Probiotics and Supplements:

- Introduce probiotics to restore the balance of healthy gut bacteria. Yogurt, kefir, or high-quality probiotic supplements can aid in re-establishing gut health.

- Explore supplements with antifungal properties like grapefruit seed extract, caprylic acid, or oil of oregano. However, always consult a healthcare professional before supplementing.

Hydration and Detoxification:

- Drink plenty of water to flush out toxins and support detoxification processes in the body.
- Herbal teas like chamomile or dandelion root can aid in liver detoxification, supporting candida treatment.

Chapter 4: Dietary Strategies for Candida Control

4.1 Anti-candida Diet: Foods to Include and Avoid

The best diet to keep Candida overgrowth to a minimum is one that is high in healthy protein, fats, and complex carbohydrates. Here are my top five food groups for beating Candida:

Protein: Protein from animal sources such as chicken, fish, shellfish, eggs

Protein from non-animal sources such as beans, legumes (such as red or brown lentils), nuts, and seeds (except peanuts and pistachios)

Fresh Vegetables: Especially dark leafy greens such as spinach, cabbage, kale and collards.

Root vegetables such as carrots and potatoes can be eaten in moderation but beware as they contain carbohydrates that will turn to sugar once eaten. Frozen, canned or jarred vegetables can be eaten but should be consumed in moderation – in general fresh is always best.

Fresh Fruits: 1-2 servings of fresh fruit per day will provide good fiber, vitamins and minerals. However, if you notice symptoms of gas, bloating and brain fog after eating fruit you may be sensitive to it and should eliminate it from your diet as well.

Complex Carbohydrates: Some people can handle having whole grains in their diet. If you find you get gas, bloating, stomach pain, blood sugar crashes or weight concerns after eating whole grains then you will need to avoid them.

Otherwise, you may be able to consume grains such as:

- Oats
- Barley
- Kamut
- Brown or wild rice
- Millet
- Teff
- Buckwheat
- Quinoa

High Quality Oils (Good Fats): All our cells have an outer layer of fat that makes up the cell membrane. When we eat high-quality oils these membranes are healthier and work optimally. When our cell membranes are working properly then we are healthier and have more energy. Unrefined and cold-pressed oils are the best when available. Good fats include (but are not limited to):

- Coconut oil
- Olive oil (avoid olives themselves as they are pickled in a brine so fall under the fermented foods category and should be avoided)
- Avocados & avocado oil
- Sunflower oil
- Safflower oil
- Fish Oil
- Flaxseed oil
- Chia Seed

4.2 Recipes and Meal Plan for Candida Control

One of the hardest things on the anti Candida Diet is figuring out exactly what to eat. You have the lists of foods to eat and avoid, but how do you make a meal out of all these new ingredients?

In this section, we've put together a fantastic range of easy and delicious recipes that are ALL compatible with your candida cleanse.

Breakfast

It's the most important meal of the day, so it should be good! A wholesome breakfast should consist of healthy fats, protein and vegetables – such as Avocado Baked Eggs with Vegetable Hash. These nutrients are essential for supporting hormonal signaling and improving your energy and mood. When you wake up in the morning, your cortisol levels should be at their highest. Cortisol is a stress hormone – but it's necessary for waking you up and keeping you alert. Eating on a regular schedule is important for keeping cortisol levels consistent and supporting early-morning energy levels.

Lunch

Lunch on the Candida diet should be as nutritionally balanced and enjoyable as any meal. An easy way to help build a balanced lunch is to include the major nutrients: protein and fiber. Asian Chicken and Cabbage Salad is perfect! Fiber isn't just necessary for keeping you regular, it keeps your blood sugar levels steady and even lowers cholesterol levels. That's why naturopaths and registered dietitians recommend getting in at least five grams of fiber at each meal. Fiber keeps you satisfied throughout the rest of the day, so you don't suffer the '3pm slump' that has you reaching for the chocolate biscuits! These fantastic lunches contain plenty of both fiber and protein to help keep you full and fueled all afternoon. And they're so delicious, you'll be looking forward to lunch break every day!

Dinner

Dinner can be tricky. Overeating – or eating the wrong kinds of food – can upset your sleep, while a dinner that doesn't satisfy can lead to reaching for a sugary late-night snack!
An ideal dinner features a balance of vegetables, protein, fiber and healthy fat. Nourishing dinner ideas like Curried Chicken Bowl are bound to make you popular at home!

Snacks

There's no harm in snacking between meals – if you do it right. Healthy snacks like Mediterranean Zucchini Dip will tide you over to your next meal without upsetting your anti-Candida protocol.

Desserts

Who said desserts were off-limits? It's natural to crave a sweet treat every now and then. The trick is to satisfy that craving without giving in to sugar. Fortunately, there are lots of natural sweeteners that contain zero sugar and don't affect your blood sugar, such as stevia, xylitol, and monk fruit extract. Fabulous desserts like Coconut Ginger Clouds use these sweeteners along with nutritious foods like coconut, avocado and healthy flours that won't ruin your good work.

Drinks

Alcohol may be out of the picture, but healthy drinks are very much encouraged. Juicing can be an excellent way to supplement your body with lots of nutrients all at once, and smoothies are an easy and delicious way to eat on the go. These drink recipes make the most of antifungal ingredients and still taste amazing.

Chapter 5: Lifestyle Adjustments for Candida Management

5.1 Stress Management Techniques

Stress can significantly impact candida overgrowth, weakening the immune system and disrupting the body's balance. Incorporating effective stress management techniques is very important in supporting candida control and overall well-being. Here are the techniques to explore:

Mindfulness Meditation: Practice mindfulness meditation to center your thoughts and reduce stress. This involves focusing on the present moment, observing thoughts without judgment, and promoting relaxation.

Deep Breathing Exercises: Engage in deep breathing exercises to alleviate stress. Take slow, deep breaths, inhaling deeply through your nose and exhaling slowly through your mouth. This simple practice helps calm the nervous system.

Yoga and Stretching: Embrace yoga or gentle stretching exercises. These practices not only ease physical tension but also promote mental relaxation, reducing stress levels.

Regular Exercise Routine: Engage in regular physical activity. Exercise releases endorphins, the body's natural stress relievers, contributing to a more positive mood and reduced stress levels.

Time Management and Prioritization: Organize your tasks and prioritize effectively. Breaking tasks into manageable chunks and setting realistic goals can reduce feelings of overwhelm and stress.

Relaxation Techniques: Explore relaxation techniques like progressive muscle relaxation or guided imagery. These methods help relax the body and mind, alleviating stress.

Adequate Sleep and Rest: Ensure you get sufficient sleep and prioritize rest. Quality sleep is vital for stress reduction and overall health. Establish a bedtime routine to promote better sleep.

Healthy Lifestyle Habits: Adopt healthy lifestyle habits such as maintaining a balanced diet, staying hydrated, and avoiding excessive caffeine or alcohol intake. A nourished body is better equipped to handle stress.

5.2 Sleep, Exercise and Other Lifestyle Factors

Beyond stress management techniques, incorporating specific lifestyle adjustments plays a vital role in managing candida overgrowth. Let's delve into the significance of sleep, exercise, and other lifestyle factors in candida management:

Quality Sleep for Healing: Adequate and quality sleep is crucial for overall health and immune function. Establishing a consistent sleep schedule and ensuring 7-9 hours of uninterrupted sleep supports your body's healing processes, aiding in candida control.

Regular Exercise and Physical Activity: Like we earlier discussed, Incorporating regular physical activity into your routine not only boosts the immune system but also helps regulate hormones and reduces stress. Aim for a mix of cardio, strength training, and flexibility exercises to support overall well-being.

Limiting Alcohol and Caffeine: Alcohol and caffeine consumption can disrupt gut health and weaken the immune system, potentially exacerbating candida overgrowth. Moderation or reduction in consumption may benefit overall health and candida management.

Hygiene and Personal Care Practices: Maintain proper hygiene to prevent the spread of candida. Practice good oral hygiene, wear breathable clothing, and avoid excessive moisture in susceptible areas to minimize candida growth.

Balancing Hormones: Hormonal imbalances can contribute to candida overgrowth. Seek ways to balance hormones through lifestyle changes, nutrition, and, if necessary, consultation with a healthcare provider.

Avoiding Environmental Triggers: Identify and minimize exposure to environmental triggers that may contribute to candida overgrowth, such as exposure to mold, chemicals, or allergens that can compromise immune function.

Chapter 6: Natural Remedy and Supplements

Treating a fungal infection can be difficult, but nature is well-equipped with natural remedies capable of accomplishing the task. Some plants contain active compounds in them that demonstrate anti-fungal properties.Below are anti-fungal herbs for killing the Candida fungus:

Oregon Grape Root: Oregon grape (Mahonia aquifolium), also known as holly-leaved barberry, is a species of flowering plant in the family Berberidaceae, native to western North America. Oregon grape root has powerful antifungal properties. It is one of the strongest antifungal herbs and one of the best herbs for candidiasis specifically. This herb may play an important role as an herbal remedy for helping with candida infection (candidiasis). Oregon grape root is one great herb for Candida infections because it contains powerful antifungal agents like berberine. In numerous studies, berberine extract has been shown to have significant antimicrobial activity against bacteria, viruses, protozoa, fungi, and yeasts. Studies have also shown that berberine has a significant antifungal effect against the Candida albicans strain in particular, which is the most common type of Candida leading to infection in humans. This makes Oregon grape root one of the best herbal remedies for treating Candidiasis.

Goldenseal Root: Goldenseal (Hydrastis canadensis)is a perennial herb in the buttercup family Ranunculaceae, native to the Eastern United States and Canada. Like Oregon grape root, goldenseal root is also high in the chemical compound berberine, an alkaloid with antibiotic and antifungal activity that has also been shown to help relieve some of the symptoms seen in people with chronic candidiasis. Like Oregan grape root, goldenseal is also a great herb for Candida.

Grape Seed Extract: Grape seed extract is derived from the ground-up seeds of red wine grapes and is available as a dietary supplement in a liquid form, tablets, or capsules. It is rich in antioxidants and has numerous health benefits. It is also powerfully antifungal. The antifungal properties of this extract make it another one of the best herbs for candidiasis and a great alternative for treating Candida and other fungal infections, especially when used in combination with diet and other anti fungal herbs.

Echinacea: Echinacea (Echinacea purpurea) is another one of the best herbs for Candida. It is native to parts of eastern North America and has a rich tradition of use by First Nations Peoples of the North American plains. It is widely known to be a powerful immune-booster, and is often used to reduce the symptoms of colds and flu. It is also traditionally used to treat fungal and bacterial infections.

Studies have shown that Echinacea targets and attacks the structure of the fungal cell wall. Fluorescence microscopy showed that yeast treated with Echinacea were significantly more prone to cell wall damage than non-treated cells. The study concluded that there was compelling evidence that the fungal cell wall is a target of Echinacea extracts and Echinacea may therefore be an effective herbal medicine in treating mycoses (fungal infections). The medicinal benefits of plants are mostly attributed to their active compounds. The active components of the Echinacea species include polysaccharides, glycoproteins, alkamides and cichoric acid, a derivative of caffeic acid. While the polysaccharides and glycoproteins are often attributed to Echnacea's immune-enhancing properties, it is the alkamides within Echinacea that appear to exert the antifungal activity of disrupting the fungal cell wall/membrane complex. All of these incredible properties make Echinacea another one of our recommended picks for the top herbs for candidiasis.

Cloves: Cloves are the flower buds of the clove tree, an evergreen also known as Syzygium aromaticum. These aromatic flower buds are often used as a culinary spice, but they also have strong antiparasitic, antibacterial and antifungal properties making them a great Candida herb. One study published in the National Library of Medicine observed the antifungal activities of clove and its volatile vapor against dermatophytic fungi. It was observed that cloves had significant antifungal activity against Candida albicans, Epidermophyton floccosum. Microsporum audouinii, Trichophyton mentagrophytes, and Trichophyton rubrum. It was shown that cloves strongly inhibit spore germination and mycelial growth of the dermatophytic fungi that were tested. The volatile vapor of clove essential oil showed fungistatic (inhibits the growth of fungi) activity whereas direct application of clove oil showed fungicidal (kills fungi) activity. Cloves contain a powerful aromatic oil called Eugenol. In vitro, eugenol has been shown to have antibacterial, antifungal, antioxidant and antineoplastic activity. Eugenol and clove extracts have also been proposed to be beneficial for gastrointestinal complaints such as nausea, diarrhea, abdominal pain and for cough, phlegm and chest congestion (as an expectorant).

Ginger: Ginger (Zingiber officinale) is a flowering plant whose rhizome, ginger root or ginger, is widely used as a spice and herbal medicine. Ginger has been used for thousands of years as an herbal remedy and it has numerous health benefits, especially for the gastrointestinal tract. Ginger also contains compounds that exhibit strong antifungal properties.

Ginseng: Ginseng (Panax ginseng) is the root of plants in the genus Panax, such as Korean ginseng, South China ginseng, and American ginseng, typically characterized by the presence of the compounds ginsenosides and gintonin. Ginseng is an herbal supplement that has been used for centuries in Chinese medicine. It is commonly praised for its antioxidant, anti-inflammatory, and immune boosting effects. A lesser known benefit of ginseng, however, is its powerful antifungal effects. Ginsenosides, active compounds in ginseng, have fungicidal (fungi-killing) effects toward Candida albicans. Studies suggest that ginsenosides may exert antifungal activity by disrupting the structure of the fungal cell membrane.

Some other common herbs with antifungal properties include:

Garlic: A common culinary herb, garlic contains numerous health benefits and exhibits powerful antifungal activity against numerous types of fungus.

Tea Tree: A popular herbal antifungal, tea tree oil is used topically to treat a variety of fungal skin and nail infections.

Turmeric: This culinary spice is widely known for its anti-inflammatory properties, but a lesser known fact about turmeric is that it is also powerfully antifungal.

Black Walnut: The green hulls of black walnut contain a chemical compound called Juglone. This compound has been extensively studied for its antimicrobial activity and ability to kill a wide range of microorganisms including bacteria, protozoa, fungi, and parasites.

Aloe Vera: The gel of the aloe vera plant also contains anti-fungal properties. It can be purchased as a supplement and easily added to water. Drinking a tablespoon of aloe vera gel a day can be a very supportive natural antifungal remedy.

Basil: Another common culinary plant, basil also helps to kill fungi and treat fungal infections. It is also delicious and easy to add to a variety of foods.

Cinnamon: This spice contains small amounts of eugenol, which is the same oil that gives cloves its powerful antifungal effects.

Lavender: This aromatic herb contains many antibacterial and antifungal properties. The oil of lavender is often applied topically to soothe and help treat fungal skin infections.

Consuming these herbs in food or applying them topically on infected areas can offer great support during a Candida elimination protocol.

Chapter 7: Candida and Gut Health

7.1 Understanding the Gut Microbiome

A biome is a distinct ecosystem characterized by its environment and its inhabitants. Your gut — inside your intestines — is in fact a miniature biome, populated by trillions of microscopic organisms. These microorganisms include over a thousand species of bacteria, as well as viruses, fungi and parasites. Your gut microbiome is unique to you. Infants inherit their first gut microbes during vaginal delivery or breastfeeding (chestfeeding). Later, your diet and other environmental exposures introduce new microbes to your biome. Some of these exposures can also harm and diminish your gut microbiota.

Why is the Gut Microbiome Important?

Most of the microorganisms in our guts have a symbiotic relationship with us, their hosts. That means we both benefit from the relationship. We provide them with food and shelter, and they provide important services for our bodies. These helpful microbes also help to keep potentially harmful ones in check.

You can think of your gut microbiome as a diverse native garden that you rely on for nutritious foods and medicines. When your garden is healthy and thriving, you thrive, too. But if the soil is depleted or polluted, or if pests or weeds are overrunning the helpful plants, it can upset your whole ecosystem.

Where is Your Gut Microbiome?

Your "gut" roughly refers to your gastrointestinal (GI) tract. Most people use it to mean your intestines. You have some gut microbiota in your stomach and small intestine, but most of them are in your large intestine (colon). They float around inside or attach to the mucous lining on the inner walls (mucosa).

The types of gut bacteria that live in your colon are different from the types that live elsewhere. They're mostly anaerobic bacteria that require a low-oxygen environment to survive. The higher oxygen, faster movement and strong digestive juices in your upper GI tract prevent them from colonizing there.

Anaerobic gut bacteria perform important functions within your colon that only they can. They help break down indigestible fibers in your digestive tract and produce essential nutrients that you can't get otherwise. By the same token, these organisms are only helpful to you within their natural microbiome.

If these bacteria stray beyond your colon, they can be harmful. Colon bacteria that manage to creep up and settle in your small intestine can interfere with digestive processes there. Colon bacteria that invade your colon wall, or that escape through a wound in your colon wall, can cause an infection in your body.

7.2 Restoring Gut Health for Candida Control

The health of your gut plays a crucial role in managing candida overgrowth. Restoring balance in the gut microbiome is key to controlling candida and promoting overall wellness. Let's explore strategies to foster a healthier gut environment:

Probiotics for Gut Balance: Introduce probiotics into your routine to support a healthy gut microbiome. Probiotics replenish beneficial bacteria, aiding in restoring balance and crowding out harmful yeast like candida. Incorporate probiotic-rich foods or high-quality supplements.

Prebiotics to Feed Beneficial Bacteria: Include prebiotic-rich foods in your diet. These foods nourish and stimulate the growth of beneficial bacteria in the gut. Options like garlic, onions, asparagus, and bananas are excellent sources of prebiotics.

Fiber-Rich Diet: Opt for a fiber-rich diet to support gut health. Fiber aids in digestion and promotes a healthy gut environment by supporting regular bowel movements. Consume a variety of fruits, vegetables, whole grains, and legumes.

Eliminating Trigger Foods: Identify and eliminate trigger foods that exacerbate gut imbalances. Processed foods, high-sugar items, refined carbohydrates, and allergens can fuel candida growth. Steer clear of these to create an inhospitable environment for candida.

Gut-Healing Supplements: Consider supplements that promote gut healing. Glutamine, aloe vera, and certain herbs like slippery elm may aid in healing the gut lining, reducing inflammation, and supporting gut integrity.

Avoiding Overuse of Antibiotics: Minimize unnecessary use of antibiotics as they disrupt the natural balance of gut bacteria. When prescribed, discuss probiotic supplementation with your healthcare provider to mitigate potential disruptions.

Periodic Detoxification and Cleansing: Engage in periodic detoxification and cleansing programs. These programs can assist in flushing out toxins and supporting the body's natural detoxification pathways, contributing to gut health.

Stress Reduction for Gut Health: Manage stress levels as stress can impact gut health. Engage in stress-relieving activities like yoga, meditation, or hobbies to support a healthier gut environment.

Chapter 8: Long-term Strategies and Preventive Measures

8.1 Maintaining Candida Free Health

One of the most important aspects of maintaining a candida-free life is avoiding sugary foods and drinks. Candida thrives on sugar, so by avoiding sugary foods and drinks, you can help to starve the candida and keep it under control. This includes not only obvious sources of sugar like candy and soda, but also less obvious sources like fruit juices, white bread, and pasta. In addition to avoiding sugar, you should also focus on eating plenty of fresh vegetables, which can help to keep your gut microbiome balanced and healthy.

Another key aspect of maintaining a candida-free life is making sure to get enough probiotics. Probiotics are live bacteria that can help to keep your gut microbiome balanced and healthy. You can get probiotics from foods like yogurt, kimchi, and sauerkraut, or you can take a probiotic supplement. In addition to probiotics, you should also make sure to get enough prebiotics. Prebiotics are the food that probiotics need to thrive, and they can be found in foods like onions, garlic, and leek. Also, stress levels can have a negative impact on the gut microbiome, making it more susceptible to candida overgrowth. Therefore, it's important to find ways to manage stress, whether that's through exercise, meditation, or simply taking some time for yourself. Also, make sure to get enough sleep! A lack of sleep can also negatively impact the gut microbiome.

8.2 Preventive Measures for Candida Recurrence

Preventing candida from coming back involves simple but essential steps to maintain your health. Here are some easy ways to make sure candida doesn't return:

Eat a Variety of Foods: Don't limit yourself to just a few types of foods. Try different fruits, vegetables, nuts, and seeds. Having lots of different foods in your diet helps your body stay strong against candida.

Manage Stress in a Healthy Way: Find ways to handle stress. Doing things like deep breathing, taking short breaks, or practicing mindfulness can help you feel better and keep your body strong.

Feed Your Gut Well: Support your gut health by eating foods like garlic, onions, and chicory. These foods help the good bacteria in your gut stay healthy and fight off candida.

Make Small Healthy Changes: Do little things every day that make you healthier. Take the stairs, get outside for fresh air, or take short walks. These small changes can add up to make you feel better.

Spend Time Outdoors: Try to get outside more often. Being in nature, getting sunlight, and fresh air can help you feel good both mentally and physically.

Try Relaxing Activities: Consider doing things like yoga or tai chi. These activities not only help your body move better but also help you feel more relaxed.

Pay Attention to Your Health: Keep an eye on your health. Talk to your doctor about what's important for your body. Checking in with your health regularly is a smart way to stay healthy.

Do Things That Make You Happy: Do things you enjoy, like painting, writing, or anything creative. These activities can help you feel better and reduce stress.

Stay Positive: Try to think about the good things in life. Being positive can help your body stay strong and healthy.

Chapter 9: Candida and Mental Health

9.1 Exploring the Connection Between Candida and Mental Well-being

If you are depressed while you suffer from regular yeast infections, or athletes foot, or have taken antibiotics recently, there is a connection. Our brains are inextricably tied to our gastrointestinal tract and our mental well being is dependent on healthy intestines. Depression, bipolar disorder, anxiety, and a host of other mental illness from autism to ADHD can be caused by an imbalance of gut microbes like fungi, and "bad" bacteria.

Candida is the opportunistic flora that typically takes over our colon with conventional diets.

Along with it comes other fungi, harmful bacteria, and parasites. An intestinal system infected with this kind of ecosystem cannot process and assimilate many of the vitamins we need, like B vitamins, which are imperative for brain function and found to be low (especially B6) in virtually anyone experiencing depression. Candida also breaks down the intestinal wall and leeches into the bloodstream, allowing other toxic byproducts to leak from the colon to the bloodstream.

Much of the body's hormone production occurs in the intestinal tract. 90 to 95% of our serotonin, the key neurotransmitter responsible for regulating mood, is produce inside our intestines. When the candida population reaches a certain point, it suppresses the production of neurotransmitters such as serotonin. A lack of serotonin leads to depression, anxiety, and other mental health problems.

Acetaldehyde, a byproduct of yeast (candida), also reacts with the dopamine neurotransmitter, which can cause mental problems such as anxiety, depression, poor concentration, and feeling spaced-out.

Candida impairs the liver's ability to store vitamin B12. We don't need much B12, but if we are low, depression and other more serious mental issues well develop quickly.

The byproducts of candida's metabolism are toxic to us. Candida goes through the bloodstream and finds other areas of the body to make home in, invading everywhere it can and making detoxifying the blood every difficult for the body. The blood becomes sluggish with diminished regenerative capacities, and the body begins to age, ache, and develop allergies and then autoimmune issues, which all lead to and fuel depression.

It's rare to find a person who suffers from depression and does not suffer from an overgrowth of candida. On the other hand, it's rare to find a person in our modern culture that does not suffer from an overabundance of candida. That said, it's very difficult to improve one's mindset without a healthy mind. And you cannot have a healthy mind without a healthy colon.

Poor colon health does lead to poor brain health, as well as poor health within the rest of the body. For almost every major disease, both physical and mental, one of the most important things you can do, and the first thing that should be done, is to improve the health of the intestinal tract by killing excess candida and balancing the gut flora. A great way to do this is with thorough detoxification.

9.2 Strategies for Balancing Mood and Emotional Health

Emotional health is an important part of your overall health. People who are emotionally healthy are in control of their thoughts, feelings, and behaviors. They're able to cope with life's challenges. They can keep problems in perspective and bounce back from setbacks. They feel good about themselves and have good relationships.

Being emotionally healthy doesn't mean you're happy all the time. It means you're aware of your emotions. You can deal with them, whether they're positive or negative. Emotionally healthy people still feel stress, anger, and sadness, but they know how to manage their negative feelings. They can tell when a problem is more than they can handle on their own. They also know when to seek help from their doctor.

Research shows that emotional health is a skill. There are steps you can take to balance your mood and emotional health.

Be Aware of Your Emotions and Reactions: Notice what in your life makes you sad, frustrated, or angry. Try to address or change those things.

Express Your Feelings in Appropriate Ways: Let people close to you know when something is bothering you. Keeping feelings of sadness or anger inside adds to stress. It can cause problems in your relationships at home, work, or school.

Think Before You Act: Give yourself time to think and be calm before you say or do something you might regret.

Manage Stress: Learn methods to cope with stress. These could include deep breathing, meditation, and exercise.

Take Care of Your Physical Health: Exercise regularly, eat healthy meals, and get enough sleep. Don't abuse drugs or alcohol. Try to keep your physical health from affecting your emotional health.

Connect with Others: Make a lunch date, join a new group, or say hi to strangers. We need positive connections with other people.

Find Purpose and Meaning: Figure out what's important to you in life, and focus on that. This could be your work, your family or friends, volunteering, caregiving, or something else. Spend time doing what feels meaningful to you.

Stay Positive: Focus on the good things in your life. Forgive yourself for making mistakes and forgive others. Spend time with healthy, positive people.

Chapter 10: Candida in Women's Health

10.1 Candida and Women's Reproductive Health

Candidiasis is one of the most common types of infections affecting women's reproductive health. It is caused by an overgrowth of the Candida fungus, which is naturally present in the body but can quickly multiply under certain conditions.

Symptoms of candidiasis include intense itching, swelling, and redness around the vulva, painful urination, and a thick, white, cottage cheese-like discharge. These symptoms may vary in severity, and some women may not experience any noticeable symptoms at all.

There are several factors that can increase the risk of developing candidiasis. These include hormonal changes, such as those during pregnancy or menopause, taking certain medications like antibiotics or steroids, having a weakened immune system, and having uncontrolled diabetes.

Treatment for candidiasis typically involves antifungal medication, which can be taken orally or applied topically to the affected area. Preventative measures that can reduce the risk of developing candidiasis include wearing loose-fitting and breathable clothing, avoiding tight-fitting undergarments, practicing good hygiene, and avoiding douching or using scented hygiene products.

It is important to seek medical attention if you experience any symptoms of candidiasis, as untreated infections can lead to complications such as chronic pain, infertility, and an increased risk for sexually transmitted infections. Taking prompt action and practicing good preventative measures can help keep women's reproductive health in optimal condition.

10.2 Managing Candida-Related Issues in Women

Candida overgrowth can pose unique challenges for women's health. Let's explore practical ways to manage candida-related issues specific to women:

Recognizing Vaginal Candidiasis Symptoms: Be aware of symptoms of vaginal candidiasis, such as itching, burning, unusual discharge, and discomfort during urination or intercourse. Understanding these signs helps in timely identification and management.

Practice Good Genital Hygiene: Maintain proper genital hygiene by using mild, unscented soaps and avoiding douching. Wear breathable cotton underwear and avoid tight-fitting clothing to promote a healthy vaginal environment.

Adopting an Anti-Candida Diet: Follow an anti-candida diet rich in whole foods, low in sugar and refined carbs. Emphasize probiotic-rich foods like yogurt or kefir to support healthy vaginal flora.

Natural Remedies for Relief: Consider natural remedies like probiotic suppositories or tea tree oil as complementary measures for managing vaginal candidiasis. However, consult a healthcare provider before using these remedies.

Seeking Medical Guidance: Consult a healthcare professional if experiencing recurrent or severe symptoms. A healthcare provider can accurately diagnose and recommend appropriate treatments, which may include antifungal medications or creams.

Addressing Hormonal Influences: Understand the link between hormonal changes and candida overgrowth. Hormonal fluctuations, such as those occurring during pregnancy or while taking birth control, can contribute to candida issues. Discuss options with a healthcare provider to manage these influences.

Managing Candida During Pregnancy: Pregnant women should seek guidance from healthcare providers when managing candida. The hormonal changes during pregnancy may increase the risk of vaginal candidiasis, and it's essential to address it safely.

Preventive Measures for Candida Control: Implement preventive measures by practicing safe sex, maintaining a healthy lifestyle, and attending routine gynecological check-ups. These steps help manage and reduce the risk of candida-related issues in women's health.

Chapter 11: Candida in Men's Health

11.1 Candida Concerns Specific to Men

You may think of yeast infections as something that only occurs in people with vaginas. But people with penises can get yeast infections too. A male yeast infection is a yeast infection that affects your penis. The medical term for yeast infections that affect men is Candida balanitis. Candida is a type of yeast that causes yeast infections. Balanitis is inflammation or an infection of the head of your penis (glans penis). Your skin has many forms of yeast that live on it, including Candida. In healthy people, this ordinarily doesn't cause any problems. But when there's an overgrowth of Candida, it can dig below the surface of your skin. This can cause a rash or skin infection. Candida grows and thrive in moist, warm environments. It's commonly found in damp, creased areas such as the foreskin of your penis.

Symptoms of a male yeast infection include pain, swelling and redness in your groin area. The redness is usually in patches. Other symptoms may include:

- Burning, itching and irritation around the head of your penis and under your foreskin.
- Thick, white discharge that resembles cottage cheese.
- Foul-smelling discharge.
- Difficulty pulling back your foreskin.
- Shiny sores or blisters on your penis.

After having a yeast infection, you may notice your skin peeling. The infection makes your skin more vulnerable. This can make it flaky or crusty and eventually it may start peeling.

Candida balanitis most commonly occurs in uncircumcised people. Other conditions and risk factors that allow Candida to grow include:

- Poor hygiene.
- Using harsh soaps.
- Not rinsing soap off your foreskin completely.
- Not drying off thoroughly.
- Irritated or damaged skin.
- Sex partners with vaginal yeast infections.

Yeast infections are more common in certain groups of people. This includes people who:

- Have a condition that weakens your immune system, such as diabetes, cancer or HIV/AIDS.

- are overweight or obese.

- Are taking antibiotics. *Antibiotics kill bacteria that normally live in your body.

- Have a sexually transmitted infection (STI).

11.2 Strategies for Men's Candida Management

Good Genital Hygiene Practices: Maintain proper genital hygiene by gently cleaning the genital area with mild, unscented soap and drying thoroughly. Avoid using perfumed products or tight-fitting clothing that can create a conducive environment for candida growth.

Dietary Adjustments for Candida Control: Adopt dietary changes that discourage candida growth. Focus on a low-sugar, anti-candida diet rich in whole foods and probiotic-rich items like yogurt or fermented foods to support overall gut health.

Natural Remedies and Hygiene Measures: Consider natural remedies such as tea tree oil-based topical applications or probiotic supplements to support healthy flora. However, consult with a healthcare provider before using these remedies for candida management.

Seeking Professional Guidance: Consult a healthcare professional if experiencing persistent or severe symptoms. Proper diagnosis by a healthcare provider ensures appropriate treatment, which may include antifungal creams or medications.

Lifestyle Adjustments for Candida Control: Manage lifestyle factors that may contribute to candida overgrowth, such as excessive stress, poor dietary choices, or antibiotic use. Adopting stress management techniques and making healthier lifestyle choices can aid in candida management.

Partners' Candida Management: Acknowledge the potential for candida transmission between partners. If one partner is managing candida issues, it's advisable for both to practice preventive measures and seek guidance if symptoms arise.

Preventive Measures for Long-term Control: Implement preventive measures to control candida issues. Maintain good overall health, practice safe sex, and prioritize regular check-ups to manage and reduce the risk of candida-related concerns.

Chapter 12: Candida and Skin Health

12.1 Understanding Candida's Impact on Skin Conditions

Candida, a naturally occurring yeast, can significantly impact skin health, causing a range of conditions and discomfort. Understanding how candida affects the skin is crucial for proper diagnosis, treatment, and prevention. Let's explore the ways in which candida influences various skin conditions:

Fungal Skin Infections: Candida can cause fungal skin infections, resulting in conditions like candidiasis. These infections typically manifest as red, itchy rashes in warm and moist areas of the body, such as folds of skin, under breasts, groin, or between fingers and toes.

Diaper Rash in Infants: In infants, candida may contribute to diaper rash. The warm, moist environment in diapers creates an ideal setting for candida growth, resulting in redness, irritation, and discomfort for the baby.

Intertrigo and Skin Folds Infections: Intertrigo, a condition affecting skin folds, can also be linked to candida overgrowth. Moisture buildup in skin folds provides an environment conducive to candida, resulting in red, raw, and often painful areas.

Nail and Cuticle Infections: Candida can affect nails and cuticles, leading to fungal nail infections (onychomycosis) or paronychia, a painful condition causing redness and swelling around the nail.

Oral Thrush and Skin Lesions: In some cases, candida can cause oral thrush, a condition characterized by white patches in the mouth. Skin lesions may also occur due to candida, especially in individuals with weakened immune systems.

Psoriasis and Eczema Aggravation: While not the primary cause, candida overgrowth may exacerbate existing skin conditions like psoriasis and eczema, leading to increased redness, itching, and discomfort.

Athlete's Foot and Jock Itch: Candida can contribute to fungal infections like athlete's foot (tinea pedis) and jock itch (tinea cruris). These infections cause itching, redness, and peeling of the affected skin areas.

Healing and Prevention: Treating candida-related skin conditions involves antifungal treatments, topical creams, and maintaining proper hygiene in affected areas. Prevention focuses on keeping skin dry, clean, and avoiding environments that promote yeast growth.

12.2 Natural Remedies and Skin Care for Candida-Related Skin Issues

Many fungi that cause these infections are largely resistant to antibiotics and other forms of medications. Fungal infections are often hard to treat and might take a while to vanish completely. Although you can easily find over-the-counter medicines and antifungal ointments in the market, most fungal skin infections can be treated with natural remedies. Let's see how to treat fungal infection on the skin naturally:

Use Tea Tree Oil: This is an antifungal and antibacterial portion that offers quick results. Mix this herbal potion with any carrier oil, like coconut oil or olive oil. Once the mixture is ready, carefully apply it over the infected area. Tea tree oil is known to stimulate the growth of new cells and hence, holds promise. Make sure you apply the mixture only on the damaged area of your skin, as the careless application might allow the fungus to spread.

Apply Honey: Raw honey is well-known for its amazing healing properties. Unpasteurised honey effectively kills bacteria and fungus as it naturally contains antiseptic hydrogen peroxide. To treat the infected spot on your skin, apply a tablespoon of honey to that region. Not only is it necessary to follow the correct remedy, but even the way the remedy is used affects the rate of recovery.

Use Coconut Oil: Coconut is another effective ingredient for skin care and healing ailments. An age-old remedy for curing skin infections, coconut oil has antifungal properties which kill fungal cells. Coconut oil, in its unheated form, is a potent antifungal agent. You can easily apply it over the infected skin area, thus making it a safe topical medicine. As it's without any side effects and is easy on the skin, it is effective for treating scalp ringworm as well. Use it thrice a day for the best results.

Use Turmeric: If you are thinking, 'how can I treat fungal skin infection naturally,' then turmeric is the answer to that question as it's the most commonly used remedy for any skin ailment. This spice has effective antimicrobial and anti-inflammatory properties. Mix it with some amount of water and apply it to the infected area. For benefits in the internal body environment, have it with warm water or rather have turmeric tea. This is the easiest home remedy for fungal infections as turmeric is found in the kitchens of all Indian households.

Garlic: Another very potent antifungal and antimicrobial herb is garlic. Those who have it as part of their diet are less susceptible to contracting fungal infections. Make a paste by crushing a handful of garlic pieces and mixing that with olive oil. Apply on the infected region for 30 minutes. Garlic helps treat ringworm, Candida, Trichophyton, Torulopsis, and Cryptococcus.

Neem Leaves: Scientifically known as Azadirachta indica, neem is a powerful fungal infection treatment. Some researchers even claim it to be the ultimate remedy. It has antifungal and natural detoxifying properties, which helps eliminate pathogens and dermophytes from the skin. Boil a handful of leaves and drink that water or apply them as a paste by thoroughly mashing them. For more effective results, neem water can be used when bathing.

Apply Aloe Vera: Aloe vera is commonly used for soothing the skin. It is considered one of the best natural home remedies for skin ailments and is an excellent healing agent for various fungal infections. Due to its antiseptic nature, aloe vera kills fungus and bacteria. It can also slow down the growth of yeast.

Use Apple Cider Vinegar: This acidic ingredient is an effective home remedy for fungal infections, rich in nutrients such as magnesium, potassium, and phosphorus and filled with antibacterial and antifungal properties. The acidic properties of apple cider vinegar slow down fungal growth, thus treating your infections quickly and effectively. Apple cider vinegar can be used in multiple ways to ward off fungal infections. Mix 2 tablespoons in warm water and drink it or dip a cotton ball in it and dab that over your skin. Doing this thrice a day will produce beneficial results.

Consume Yoghurt: Yoghurt and other probiotics contain a considerable amount of good bacteria, which help keep fungal infections at bay. These fight microbes that cause such infections. Another great source of probiotics is fermented food. But in case these aren't working, you can take probiotic supplements which have a concentrated dosage of good bacteria.

Use Lemongrass Oil: Lemongrass is another ingredient laden with excellent antimicrobial properties. Mix lemongrass oil with a carrier oil and dab it gently on the affected area with a cotton ball or swab twice a day for best results.

Chapter 13: Candida in Children and Infants

13.1 Candida in Pediatric Health

Candida infections in children most commonly in the mouth, also known as oral thrush or thrush, are common in infants and toddlers. Thrush can also affect the nails, eyes, and skin folds in the neck and armpits, as well as the diaper area, including the vagina and groin folds. Newborns and young children have certain risk factors for candida infection higher than others when:

During Labor: Infants with maternal candidiasis can occur right away. when the baby is still in the uterus, but most commonly when it passes through the vagina at birth.

Medication: Sometimes children get a candida infection after taking antibiotics. Although antibiotics fight germs that cause illness in children, they can also affect strains of "good" bacteria that help keep the symbiotic population in check. Not rinsing your mouth with water after using the inhaler can also lead to a candida infection.

Health conditions: In some children with limited health conditions, fungi can enter the bloodstream. The most at-risk of blood candida infections include infants born prematurely or with very low birth weight, children with long-term intravenous catheterization, and children with weakened immune systems due to cancer, taking medications. For these children, oral nystatin and fluconazole are often used to prevent candidiasis. If a Candida infection has progressed to become chronic or occurs in an older child's mouth, it could be a sign of a weakened immune system, such as infection with human immunodeficiency virus (HIV). A candida infection of the skin, mouth (thrush), or even vaginal candidiasis in children over 2-3 years old, can also be a sign of diabetes.

Signs and Symptoms in Children with Candidiasis

Symptoms appear to include painful white or yellow patches on the tongue, lips, gums, roof of the mouth, and inner cheeks. The fungus can also spread into the esophagus, making it painful for a child to swallow. In addition, strains of Candida on the skin can make diaper rash caused by a fungal infection worse, causing redness and sensitivity in the affected area, along with a satellite red border.

Adolescent girls with a vaginal yeast infection may have symptoms such as itching, pain, redness, and a strong-smelling vaginal discharge. Children receiving intravenous drugs Symptoms are varied in children with candidiasis during treatment with chemotherapy or long-term medications given through an intravenous catheter.

In these cases, the fungus easily enters the blood system. Once in the bloodstream, yeast can travel throughout the body, infecting the heart, lungs, livers, kidneys, eyes, brain and skin. The early signs of a candida blood-borne infection are fever and blockage of the venous catheter.

13.2 Strategies for Managing Candida in Children

Candida overgrowth in children, though challenging, can be effectively managed with specific strategies tailored to their unique needs. Here are practical approaches for parents and caregivers to address candida-related concerns in children:

Recognizing Symptoms in Children: Be vigilant for signs of candida overgrowth in children, including oral thrush (white patches in the mouth), diaper rash, persistent skin rashes, or digestive issues. Early recognition is key to prompt management.

Maintaining Good Hygiene: Ensure good hygiene practices for children. Regular diaper changes, keeping skin folds dry, and using mild, unscented products aid in preventing candida-related diaper rashes or skin infections.

Healthy Nutrition for Immune Support: Promote a balanced and nutritious diet to support their immune system. Limiting sugary snacks and processed foods helps control candida growth.

Providing Probiotics and Prebiotics: Consider incorporating probiotics and prebiotics into their diet. Probiotic-rich foods like yogurt and prebiotic sources such as bananas or oats support gut health and aid in controlling candida.

Addressing Candida in Oral Health: For oral thrush, use prescribed antifungal medications as directed by a pediatrician. Maintaining oral hygiene, such as gentle brushing of gums and teeth, is crucial.

Treating Skin Infections Promptly: If a child develops skin rashes or infections suspected to be candida-related, consult a pediatrician for proper diagnosis and treatment. Antifungal creams or ointments may be recommended.

Managing Underlying Health Conditions: Children with underlying health conditions or those on antibiotics are more prone to candida overgrowth. Ensure any medications or treatments are administered under medical supervision.

Encouraging Healthy Lifestyle Habits: Promote healthy habits like regular handwashing, sufficient sleep, and outdoor activities. These habits support overall well-being, contributing to a stronger immune system.

Seeking Professional Guidance: Consult pediatric healthcare providers for persistent or severe symptoms. Professional guidance ensures accurate diagnosis and appropriate treatment for children affected by candida overgrowth.

Chapter 14: Candida and Immune System Support

The interaction between Candida and your immune system is an important part of your Candida treatment plan. A strong immune system is your first line of defense against a Candida overgrowth, but it's also one of the first systems in your body that the Candida attacks. So not only do you need to repair your immune system from the damage that the Candida has caused, but you also need to make it even stronger to keep your Candida in check over the long run.

A weak immune system is often associated with illnesses like adrenal fatigue and leaky gut syndrome. In addition to your probiotics and antifungals, there are a number of ways to help your body cope with these illnesses and rebuild your immune system. If you take the right supplements, make a few changes in your daily routine and adopt a healthier lifestyle, your body will be able to do much of the work in beating your Candida infestation.

Supplements To Boost Your Immune System
Vitamins: Vitamin C helps with Candida overgrowth in three ways. First, it provides support to your adrenals, two small organs that are crucial for your metabolism and blood sugar regulation (as well as your body's production of things like anti-inflammatories and antihistamines). Second, Vitamin C boosts your immune system and gives your body the best chance possible to fight off the Candida yeast.

Lastly, it helps to boost your stomach acid, which slows the Candida overgrowth.

Other vitamins that can be helpful include vitamins A and E, as well as pantothenic acid (Vitamin B5). Vitamin A helps your body defeat infection by influencing the cells in certain mucosal surfaces, while studies on Vitamin E have shown it to be effective in boosting immune response after vaccinations.

Immune-Supportive Herbs: You can try some herbal remedies to reduce stress on your immune system too. In chapter 6 of this book, we discussed various herbs one can use to treat Candida, so look back.

Other Ways to Strengthen your Immune System
Cut Back on the Caffeine: Caffeine is one of the biggest causes of adrenal fatigue, and therefore

immune system weakness. It's not easy to reduce your coffee intake, so take some time to lower your daily dose. Start by cutting out your afternoon coffee or switching to decaf, then gradually reduce the weakness of your morning cup too. You can try chicory coffee as an alternative – it tastes similar, contains prebiotics to promote the rebalancing of your gut flora, and stimulates the production of healthy digestive enzymes.

Gentle Exercise: Some light exercise will improve your circulation and support your immune system. Don't overdo it though – a strenuous workout will place your body under stress and weaken your adrenals further.

Reduce Stress: Physical and emotional stress are major contributors to immune system failure, so you need to find a way to cut some of the stress out of your life. Take a week or two off work and go on a relaxing holiday if you can. Don't just think in the short term either – if you can reduce your stress levels long term that's even better.

Rest Up: One of the most important things you can do for your adrenals is take a good rest. If you can't get away on holiday, at least make sure that you go to sleep reasonably early. Staying up late is actually quite stressful on your body, so do your adrenals a favor and make sure you get your 8 hours of sleep.

If you're reading this book "Defeating Candida", you may also be interested in my book on prostate cancer and breast cancer. Tap the links above to read them.

Thank you for purchasing my book. I'd really appreciate it if you could take a moment to leave a review. Your feedback will help me improve and make my next book even better. I'm always looking forward to improving, so please do not hold back! Thank you for your time and support.

www.ingramcontent.com/pod-product-compliance
Lightning Source LLC
Chambersburg PA
CBHW070850260726
48661CB00004B/1338